Contents

Introduction

Welcome to the journey towards a healthier, more vibrant you. In the hustle and bustle of modern life, it's all too easy to neglect our well-being. We often find ourselves overwhelmed with work, family responsibilities, and the daily demands of a fast-paced world. In this whirlwind of activity, our health can take a backseat, and we might forget that true wealth begins with good health."Fit For Life" is your trusted companion on the path to lasting well-being. This comprehensive guide is designed to empower you with the knowledge and tools to take control of your physical fitness, nourish your body with wholesome nutrition, and explore the benefits of natural health remedies. It's a roadmap to help you unlock your full potential, revitalize your spirit, and embark on a lifelong journey towards optimal health and vitality.

The Three Pillars of Wellness

This book revolves around three core principles that form the foundation of a healthy and fulfilling life:

Physical Fitness: We begin by exploring the world of fitness, understanding the importance of regular exercise, and discovering how it can transform your body and mind. Whether you're a seasoned athlete or just starting your fitness journey, "Fit For Life" offers guidance for creating a tailored exercise routine that suits your needs.

Nutrition: The saying "you are what you eat" holds profound truth. In the chapters dedicated to nutrition, we delve into the essentials of balanced eating, uncover the benefits of key vitamins and minerals, and discuss dietary supplements and herbal remedies. You'll learn how to make informed choices about what you put on your plate and how it impacts your overall health.

Natural Health Remedies: Nature has provided us with an abundance of remedies to address various health concerns. "Fit For Life" introduces you to the world of herbal remedies, natural supplements, and holistic practices that can enhance your well-being. From managing stress to supporting joint health and cognitive function, you'll discover effective, safe, and evidence-based approaches to achieving optimum health.

Your Personal Wellness Journey

This book is not a one-size-fits-all solution; it's your personalized guide to wellness. "Fit For Life" encourages you to embrace a holistic approach that considers your unique needs, goals, and circumstances. Whether you're seeking to boost workout performance, manage your weight, or enhance mental clarity, this book provides the insights, practical tips, and resources to help you succeed.

Your journey towards a healthier, more vibrant life starts here. As you turn the pages of "Fit For Life," you'll find inspiration, expert advice, and actionable steps to cultivate a lifestyle that supports your well-being. Together, let's embark on a path to lasting health, vitality, and the fulfillment of your fitness and wellness aspirations.

What is Fit For Life?

Harvey Diamond's Fit for Life is a diet plan developed by Harvey and Marilyn Diamond.

The diet formula works on the concept that eating a specific combination of food promotes good health. It also prohibits eating certain types of food altogether.

The diet primarily encourages eating whole grains and gradually eliminating refined grains and other processed food from your diet.

• Advances in Nutrition – Unfortunately, this idea of eliminating refined grains may not be based on solid science. According to some research, "the recommendation to reduce refined grain intake based on results from studies linking a Western dietary pattern to numerous adverse health outcomes is contrary to a substantial body of published scientific evidence. Future research needs to better define refined grain intake to distinguish between staple grain foods and indulgent grain foods, and to better design randomized controlled trials to resolve discrepancies between results from observational studies and such trials with regard to determining the benefits of whole grains compared with refined grains."

• The American Journal of Clinical Nutrition – In one clinical study, replacing whole grains for refined grains evoked some positive changes on gut microbiota, which could be a benefit to consider.

• The American Journal of Clinical Nutrition – Another study published in this journal showed that whole grains actually affected resting metabolic rate and "may favorably influence energy balance and may help explain epidemiologic associations between whole-grain consumption and reduced body weight and adiposity."

Food and exercise are the two critical aspects of healthy living. You are what you eat, so when you decide to get Fit for Life, you should research the many diet plans currently on the market.

The Basic Ideas For Harvey Diamond Fit For Life Diet Plan

This diet is all about the good and bad combinations of food. 'Dead' food is not a part of the diet.

Diamond believed that the wrong combination of food could cause the food to 'ferment' in the stomach. Here are the main points of the diet plan.

Dairy products can cause allergies and should rarely be eaten, if at all. They are not considered to contribute valuable nutrition.

Water is not an option during meals because it would dilute digestive juices.

Fruits should be eaten raw and fresh. And you must eat them without other food.

It is ill-advised to combine proteins with carbohydrates during meals.

The dietary principle involves consuming predominantly 'live' food with high water content.

When animal protein is eaten, avoid complex carbohydrates.

Fit for Life recipes Harvey Diamond offers to let us see what this diet offers each day.

Origins

Fit for Life is the creation of Harvey and Marilyn Diamond. The diet first came to the attention of the public in the mid-1980s with the publication of the book Fit for Life, which has sold millions of copies. On the official Fit for Life website, Diamond claims that the diet "spawned juice and salad bars, fruit sellers on the streets of New York, and the juice industry." He also claims the book "launched a nutritional awakening in the United States and other Western countries."These are impressive claims for a book written by a man whose "doctoral degree" came from the American College of Life Science, a non-accredited correspondence school founded in 1982 by a high school dropout.

Diamond has appeared on dozens of television talk shows explaining his theories on how eating foods in the correct combination and avoiding the "wrong" combinations of food can bring about weight loss without calorie counting or exercise. In the 2000s, the Fit for Life system added the Personalized FFL Weight Management Program. This program uses what they call Biochemical Analyzation, Metabolic Typing and Genetic Predispositions to individualize and personalize the dietary protocols. The resulting diet is said to be effective only for one specific.

KEY TERMS

Alternative medicine —a system of healing that rejects conventional, pharmaceutical-based medicine and replaces it with the use of dietary supplements and therapies such as herbs, vitamins, minerals, massage, and cleansing diets. Alternative medicine includes well-established treatment systems such as homeopathy, Traditional Chinese Medicine, and Ayurvedic medicine, as well as more-recent, fad-driven treatments.

Cholesterol —a waxy substance made by the liver and also acquired through diet. High levels in the blood may increase the risk of cardiovascular disease.

Conventional medicine —mainstream or Western pharmaceutical-based medicine practiced by medical doctors, doctors of osteopathy, and other licensed health care professionals.

Dietary fiber —also known as roughage or bulk. Insoluble fiber moves through the digestive system almost undigested and gives bulk to stools. Soluble fiber dissolves in water and helps keep stools soft.

Dietary supplement —a product, such as a vitamin, mineral, herb, amino acid, or enzyme, that is intended to be consumed in addition to an individual's diet with the expectation that it will improve health.

Enzyme —a protein that change the rate of a chemical reaction within the body without themselves being used up in the reaction.

Mineral —an inorganic substance found in the earth that is necessary in small quantities for the body to maintain a health. Examples: zinc, copper, iron.

Naturopathic medicine —An alternative system of healing that uses primarily homeopathy, herbal medicine, and hydrotherapy and rejects most conventional drugs as toxic.

Vitamin —a nutrient that the body needs in small amounts to remain healthy but that the body cannot manufacture for itself and must acquire through diet.

individual and can be used for that person's entire life. Diamond has also begun selling nutritional supplements, many of which are strongly recommended in his newest version of the Fit for Life system.

Description

Fit for Life is a food combining diet based on the theory that to lose weight, one must not eat certain foods together. The philosophy behind the diet comes from Diamond's interest in natural hygiene, an offshoot of naturopathic medicine. In his original book, Diamond claimed that if a person ate foods in the wrong combination, they would "rot"in the stomach. He also categorized foods as "dead foods"that "clog"the body and "living foods" that cleanse the body. The newest version of Fit for Life talks less about rotting, dead, and living foods and more about "enzyme deficient foods."However, the general message about food combining is the same.

According to Diamond, dead foods are meats and starches. Living foods are raw fruits and vegetables. His diet plan requires that these foods not be eaten together. Some of the Fitness for Life rules include:

Only fruit and fruit juice should be eaten from the time one awakes until noon. Fruits cleanse the body

Fruits are good for health only if they are eaten alone.They should never be eaten with any other food

Lunch and dinner can consist of either carbohydrates and vegetables or proteins and vegetables

Carbohydrates and proteins should never be put in the stomach at the same time

No dairy foods should ever be eaten

Water should never be drunk at meals

One day each week (the same day every week) is a free day, when the individual can eat whatever he or she wants."

Function

The goal of the Fit for Life diet is to help people lose weight and keep their body healthy through diet. Diamond states that people do not gain weight because they eat too many calories and exercise too little. Instead, he considers the cause of weight gain to be eating protein-rich foods at the same time as carbohydrate-rich foods. He argues that enzymes that digest proteins interfere with enzymes that digest carbohydrates, and therefore, these two foods should not be eaten together. His program makes little mention of the role of different types of fats—saturated, unsaturated, and transfat—in diet, dietary fiber, the role of water in health, or of the need to exercise.

The Fit for Life program says it is a lifestyle program that will teach people to be healthier. Along with the personalized diet program, dieters get a "Clinical Manual"that claims to teach them how their body works, what is healthy for them, and what is not. The program is heavily infused with an alternative medicine approach to health and diet, and many of the explanations it gives for the way the body works are scientifically questionable and not accepted by practitioners of conventional medicine.

Don't Call it a Diet: "Fit For Life" Changes Everything

There are so many ways to lose weight. You can try the Beverly Hills Diet. Or eat like a cave man. Why not subsist on liquid protein alone? Or sip cold coffee throughout the day like a certain ELLE fashion assistant, who nibbles off a bit of rice cake only when he feels faint. Restrictive diets are all the rage.

With that said, crash diets rarely work for me. During a recent Master Cleanse—you know, the one where you drink nothing but water laced with maple syrup, cayenne pepper, and lemon—I undid each day of starvation with a late night bodega binge. Editor's note: Don't try this at home.

What you should try, is this new program Fit For Life, created by Harvey and Marilyn Diamond. When a friend called Harvey "Blimpo," he was inspired to ditch the punishing diets that had made him lose and just as quickly gain weight, and really change his life. Harvey's story resonates because not so long ago, my own recent weight gain was brought to light by a friend who pointed it out, publicly.

"I've never seen you eat so much," she said, as I sliced what would be my second avocado of the day in my boyfriend's kitchen. "Intimacy looks good on you." What she meant was intimacy looks heavy on you. "Don't worry, you'll lose the weight." And just like that, I realized that no, I didn't wash my jeans on high heat. The dry cleaner doesn't shrink dresses. Salt isn't to blame for my swollen face. I had simply gotten a bit fat. For me, at least.

If I wanted to go from "Blimpo" to Brooke Shields by fall, I needed a new plan. No more quick-fix fad diets. I needed something that would work longterm. Enter Fit For Life, based upon the principle that the body functions best when "natural cycles" are adhered to. Noon to 8 p.m.. is appropriation (eating and digestion), 8 p.m. to 4 a.m. is assimilation (absorption and use), 4 a.m. to noon is elimination (of waste and food). Simply put, eat and excrete at a certain time and your body will feel better forever.

There are a few key rules to living by Fit For Life, including:

Eat your water: According to Diamond, nothing, not even water itself, hydrates the body like fruits and vegetables, which should make up 70 percent of your daily intake. The other 30 percent is comprised of "concentrated foods" like nuts, grains, and lean protein. Which brings me to Diamond's next point...

Handle protein with care: Americans are obsessed with protein, but most eat too much, he says. While FFL discourages eating meat (it's often injected with hormones), lean protein is allowed in small doses when eaten alone.

Be a matchmaker: Meat and potatoes, fish and rice, cereal and milk are all bad couples, but take apart each pair, add a green vegetable, and you're Diamond-approved.

Fruit needs alone time: According to Diamond, "fruit rots and turns into acid," when combined with other food in the stomach. According to Fit For Life, fruit is for breakfast and a mid-morning snack, but after 12 p.m., fruit should only be eaten on an empty stomach, except for on all-fruit "for maximum weight loss" days.

Exercise: Just move something. Even a 20 minute walk will do.

But whatever you do, do not overeat: Do not overeat. Do not overeat. Do not overeat. Do not overeat. Do not overeat. Do not overeat. Do not overeat. Do not overeat. Do not overeat. Because everything, even vegetables can be eaten in excess, and excess leads to weight gain.

There goes my voluminous baby carrot habit. Yes, when it comes to diets, I have always gravitated to plans with some kind of "all you can eat" component. Often it's vegetables or one specific fruit. Maybe Tab or sugarless iced tea with Sweet'N Low. Sometimes, and I'm not proud of it, an entire pack of Bubble Yum. But, Diamond isn't about that binge life. He's about being fit. Here, a loose adaptation of the program.

SAMPLE DAY

I wake up with hunger pangs at 3 a.m. during "elimination hours," and justify eating a small banana. Surely this counts towards my morning fruit intake. Diamond encourages grazing on fruit throughout the morning, often eating up to three bananas.

Breakfast: Really, second breakfast: I peel another banana and prepare a bowl of ripe strawberries, sliced kiwi, and a few red grapes. I can't stop thinking about mid-morning fruit snack.

Mid-morning snack: At the office, there's a photoshoot for our November issue, which means catered food is everywhere. I avoid a plate of bagels and scoop some diced melon into a coffee cup. Instantly, I want another cup of fruit, but ELLE's photographer catches me hovered over the spread. "Just over here binging, huh Julie," he says, and I shuffle back on set with my melon cup.

Lunch: Catered lunch is sandwiches, which I mentally dissect according to Diamond's food-pairing rules. Turkey and Swiss on ciabatta is off-limits because meat and cheese don't go together. Ditto chicken with mozzarella and pesto. I settle for a portobello mushroom, zucchini, and avocado sandwich and peel the cold marinated strips from the bread. Throughout the shoot, I return to the table, gutting a total of four vegetarian sandwiches.

Fit For Life doesn't call for a mid-afternoon snack, but fruit is allowed three hours after lunch, "if you're still hungry." I go for Diet Coke and gum instead, both discouraged on the plan.

Exercise: When I finish work around 9 p.m., I'm well into assimilation and past approved eating hours, but I haven't exercised yet so it's time for the gym. I listen to the Miami Vice soundtrack and jog on the treadmill for 30 minutes and walk for 10 without really breaking a sweat.

Dinner: My easy run makes me extra hungry, but all the restaurants have closed, and I have no choice but to eat a leftover salad from my boyfriend's refrigerator. It's made of greens, roasted sweet potatoes, kidney beans, avocado, and cranberries. Do not overeat. Do not overeat. Do not overeat. Halfway in, I'm comfortably full, but I pack forkfuls of lettuce into my mouth until it's all gone. An hour later I want more food, so I tear off half of a wheat pita (Diamond says whole-wheat bread isn't so bad) and smear it with hummus. I'm pretty sure this is a match made in "no."

HOW I FEEL

Not good. Fit For Life's fruititarian days give me sugar hangovers, and on other days, I am insatiably hungry. Diamond's "do not overeat" mantra taunts me Blimpo-style, and nearly every meal on the plan evolves into a binge. With that being said, I can't argue with the appropriation, assimilation, and elimination schedule. While Fit For Life didn't help me drop the "intimacy" weight, it has changed the way I see food, at least for now.

Harvey and Marilyn Diamond developed the Fit for Life Diet in the 1980's and co-authored a book by the same name. The diet is based on the concept of proper food combining, an eating method that prohibits consuming certain types of foods together. There is much controversy surrounding this fad diet. Consult your doctor before making any major changes to your diet.

Breakfast

The Fit for Life Diet plan recommends eating carbohydrates early in the day, reserving them mainly for breakfasts and lunches. You should consume carbohydrates either alone or with vegetables, but never with fruit or animal protein foods. Examples of carbohydrate breakfast items are oatmeal, cracked wheat cereals, whole grain breads, muffins and bagels. You should eat these without butter, cream or fruit spreads. Diamond recommends consuming only whole grains and eliminating processed or refined grains from the diet completely.

Lunch

Lunch on the Fit for Life plan offers two options: combining carbohydrates with vegetables, or protein foods with vegetables. Again, the diet discourages eating carbohydrates and protein foods together. Examples of carbohydrate lunches include brown rice and sauteed vegetables, or a whole wheat pita with lettuce, bean sprouts and shredded carrots. Lunches with protein foods include salads with garbanzo beans or sunflower seeds, and lentil or three-bean soup with vegetables. You would use light oil dressings in place of cream dressings or mayonnaise.

Dinner

Protein foods are the focus of dinners on the Fit for Life diet. Diamond recommends avoiding animal proteins as much as possible, with the exception of organic eggs and fresh fish, and consuming mostly legumes and dried beans. Some possible dinner items might include meatless chili with assorted raw vegetables, stir-fried tofu and diced Asian vegetables, or broiled salmon and steamed asparagus.

Effective Fitness Supplements And Natural Health

Fit for Life: Effective Fitness Supplements and Natural Health" is a comprehensive guide that explores the world of fitness supplements and natural health remedies. This book delves into the importance of balanced nutrition, essential vitamins and minerals, herbal remedies, and protein supplements for optimal health and fitness. It also covers the benefits of pre-workout and post-workout supplements, weight management solutions, joint health, and cognitive supplements.

With a holistic approach to health and wellness, "Fit for Life" emphasizes the integration of fitness, nutrition, and natural health practices for a well-rounded lifestyle. Whether you're looking to enhance workout performance, manage weight, improve mental clarity, or support overall health, this book provides valuable insights, evidence-based information, and practical tips to help you achieve your fitness and wellness goals. Discover the power of supplements and natural remedies in achieving a healthier and more vibrant life.

Achieve good health and fitness through Fit For Life Sciences Institute's natural health courses and products. We can help you live more responsibly through alternative health methods. With our programs, you will learn about how healthy eating improves your overall health and stops certain illnesses so that you can live a happier and more stress-free lifestyle.

As a professional university extension nutritionist statewide, my primary program and responsibility is to combat misinformation and provide sound nutritional information. It's on that basis that I especially say that this book is not recommended except as a prime example of extreme food faddism.

The "Not Recommended" stamp was on a hot line book review dispatched to members of the California Dietetic Assn. by Swenerton.

Still, with 1 million copies in print, "Fit for Life" has remained No. 1 on some of the most prestigious best-seller lists longer than is the fate of most health/diet books--31 weeks on the New York Times best-seller list, and remains at the top of The Los Angeles Times list. Co-author Harvey Diamond largely credits television personality Merv Griffin for helping to rocket sales nationwide. "We really owe a lot to Merv Griffin. He's constantly talking about our book on his show."

Diamond and his wife, Marilyn, who operate the International Health Systems nutrition counseling service in Santa Monica, make no bones about having received their nutritional training from the American College of Health Science, a non-accredited college in Austin, Tex. According to Harvey Diamond, all the information upon which their theories are based comes from the field of natural hygiene. "Maybe we're not in agreement with the medical profession, but we know our program works."

Emphasis on Carbohydrates

Actually, the Diamonds' push for complex carbohydrates (fruits, vegetables and grains) over meats is not far off from the U.S. dietary guidelines for Americans, which emphasize complex carbohydrates and de-emphasize fatty meats. And the recipes in the book developed by Marilyn, who is director of the Institute for Nutritious Home Cooking in Santa Monica and does cooking demonstrations on television, are excellent and can apply to, if not enhance, any diet. The vegetable dishes are particularly appealing (stir-fried lo mein with shredded vegetables, curried vegetables and cabbage strudel).

However, it's the principal theory of the book, which had been refuted by the scientific community decades ago, that seems to grate at the craw of established nutritionists. Likc "The Beverly Hills Diet," a best-selling predecessor by Judy Mazel, "Fit for Life" is based on the principles of so-called "food combining, a turn-of-the-century notion that when combined inappropriately foods will become rotten, cannot be assimilated, toxify the body and make people fat."

The proper approach, say the Diamonds, is never to mix alkaline foods (fruits, vegetables and grains) with acidic foods (protein). For example, one never eats either starch or protein with vegetables and fruits. Sandwiches are made with vegetables since bread is a starch.

Nor does one thwart the elimination process taking place from 4 a.m. to noon each day by eating anything but fruit or juice for breakfast.

Food combining, according to the theory, cuts the digestive process by two-thirds, preventing food from remaining in the system longer than five hours, compared with up to 16 hours for some hard-to-digest foods, such as protein. For instance, the theory suggests, fruit should never be eaten with or immediately following anything. A grace period of three hours after meals is usually advised.

Furthermore, according to the theory, because protein digestion is done by enzymes that are more acidic in nature than enzymes that carry out carbohydrate digestion, these enzymes nullify one another.

"These archaic turn-of-the-century notions are totally invalid and were thoroughly refuted long ago," Swenerton said. "The mucousless diet of the turn-of-the-century suggesting that certain combinations of foods caused toxins and mucous was at a time when people knew very little about the chemistry of food and little of the basic physiology and biology of the body. These notions are in complete conflict with reliable research-based information on basic physiology and nutrition. And there is no scientific evidence to support such claims.

"What is surprising is that in these modern days with so much accurate information available in public school, or even at elementary levels, that the public would succumb to these grossly wild ideas."

However, the Diamonds, who seem sincere and full of conviction about their program, pooh-pooh the critics. "I don't care whether scientific evidence exists or not. I ask people to combine their foods for one week, then tell me how you feel. One million people are interested in it despite what the scientists think," Harvey Diamond said.

Diamond, a former wood carver at the Renaissance Faire in Agoura, who devoted his extra time to the study of natural hygiene, claims that his father's health problems seemed to have transferred themselves to the son, until Diamond stumbled on the food-combining theory. "Once I started on the program, I felt reborn. I lost my stomach aches and had a strong desire to spread the word." He began his practice as a nutrition counselor in 1973 working out of a health food store.

Although much of the nutritional information in the book has scientific basis in fact, there is, according to Swenerton, enough nonsense mingled with it to render it "nonsensical." Said Swenerton: "He has intermingled good information with bad information. He has taken sense and mixed it with nonsense, making it difficult for the reader to distinguish what is accurate and what is not."

Diamond also claims that energy is conserved by eating fruit because fruit does not digest in the stomach. "(The fruits) pass through the stomach in 20 to 30 minutes, as if they were going through a tunnel . . . this energy is automatically redirected to cleanse the body of toxic waste, thereby reducing weight," states Diamond.

Swenerton: "That's just nonsense. All foods that are ingested are broken down, whether it is fruit or any complex carbohydrate. There is no difference in energy from complex carbohydrates. The rate of digestion may be different. Simple sugars are digested more quickly than complex sugars, but neither would remove toxic wastes from within body tissues."

Some other points of departure:

"Most fruits contain ample calcium," claims Diamond, believing that the milk-drinking population has been led down the garden path. "Dietitians are dependent on the cow for calcium. If the cows get their calcium from the plant kingdom, certainly humans can, too."

According to Diamond, the body doesn't have the mechanism to break down milk and utilize it. "In nature, we don't see animals taking milk from other animals. Only human mammals insist on drinking milk of another mammal."

Questioning Established Views

The question raised about calcium in relation to milk sent abrasive sparks to established views about the role of dairy products, which provide 75% of the calcium in the American diet. Dairy products are one of the major groups of foods recommended since the outset of the Recommended Dietary Allowances in 1945 when U.S.

Department of Agriculture nutritionists created the concept of the Four Food Group system of eating for a nutritionally well-balanced diet.

Appropriate servings of vegetables and fruit, grains, meat and meat alternates and dairy products would provide all the nutrients needed by Americans for optimal health. The Diamonds claim that there are only two food groups--fruits and vegetables are one group and everything else the second group.

The Dairy Council of California, an educational arm of the dairy industry in California, had this to say about Diamond's calcium claims:

"As a nutrition education organization we're very concerned about a book like 'Fit for Life.' Scientifically, most of the information is not valid. But our real concern is that it encourages people to eliminate major groups of foods, not the least of which is dairy products, which provide nearly 75% of the calcium in the American diet," said Beverly McKee, communications coordinator of the Dairy Council of California.

Swenerton has added yet another concern about relying solely on fruits and vegetables for calcium.

"Saying that calcium in milk cannot be broken down and is unavailable to the body is scientifically incorrect," she said. "But our primary concern is that they (Diamonds) claim that a diet of fruits and vegetables with a few seeds and nuts would be adequate for a growing child and pregnant woman. We're concerned that such a restricted diet without adequate protein source and other nutrients--including calcium--would do serious harm to a developing fetus during pregnancy, and serious harm to a growing child. There simply isn't enough calcium in fruits and vegetables to provide adequate calcium to a growing body or pregnant woman and her fetus."

There is no indication in the book for any modifications in the diet for children. Pregnant women are informed that the food-combining program "fulfills all the dietary requirements for both mother and child during gestation."

"Actually, the most beneficial diet during pregnancy (and at any other time) is a diet that has a preponderance of raw fruit and vegetables, and some raw nuts and seeds. This will supply all the fuel, amino acids, minerals, fatty acids and vitamins needed to perpetuate a high level of health," says Marilyn Diamond in the book.

Dairy products provide about 300 milligrams calcium per serving, compared with 100 to 200 milligrams calcium from green leafy vegetables. Fruits and other vegetables contain less calcium, providing only 10% of the calcium in the American food supply, but can be called upon to increase total calcium intake. Only three servings from the dairy group can provide calcium requirements for adults. It would take eight to 10 servings of fruits and vegetables to provide calcium needs.

Growing teen-agers, pregnant nursing women and pregnant and nursing teen-agers require 1,200 to 1,600 milligrams calcium per day. Most adults require 800 milligrams calcium per day. However, calcium recommendations for pre-menopausal women has increased to 1,000 milligrams as a measure to prevent osteoporosis, a crippling old-age disease. (See story on latest calcium research findings on Page 2.)

Diamond claims that when food is not digested, the food then putrifies or ferments, forming toxic substances that accumulate in the body and translates into overweight problems.

"Wrong," Swenerton said. Those foods that are not digested simply are not digested and are passed out in the fecal material. They are not accumulated in the body. Non-assimilated foods are assimilated by definition. They are excreted in fecal material and can't turn into fat, as the author claims.

The primary concern, according to Swenerton, is that bits and pieces of information are erroneous, making it virtually impossible for the reader to distinguish between fact and fiction.

Diamond correctly states that the human brain burns fuel (glucose), which is readily assimilated from carbohydrates, not proteins, and that the body can transform protein to glucose through an emergency process utilized by the body when there are insufficient carbohydrates in the body.

But Diamond goes on to explain (and here the reader might have difficulty with the drift): "Flesh foods supply no fuel, no energy. Fuel is built from carbohydrates. Meat has virtually no carbohydrates. In other words, no fuel value. Fats may supply energy, but they must undergo a longer and less efficient digestive process and fats may be converted into fuel only when the body's carbohydrate reserves are depleted. . . ."

According to Swenerton, proteins are digested in a completely different part of the gastrointestinal tract than carbohydrates, so there is no physiological basis for Diamond's claim.

"Most foods naturally come with carbohydrates and proteins together. Diamond claims that those that occur separately can be digested while those that do not cannot be digested. There is a lack of understanding of the basic physiology process," she said.

Diamond also claims that flesh eaters are more apt to develop Vitamin B-12 deficiency because a substance secreted out of the stomach into another part of the body is destroyed when meat remains in the stomach, thus causing vitamin deficiency. "Most people who eat meat have Vitamin B-12 deficiency. It's not a problem for vegetarians. A million and a half Hindus don't have a problem."

Swenerton says that there is no scientific evidence to support the claim that flesh eaters develop Vitamin B-12 deficiency.

Nutritionists such as Susan Magrann, representing the California Dietetic Assn. on various subjects, thinks the deluge of diet books on the market can be confusing and difficult for consumers to assess. There are, however, certain guidelines that should help the buyer make knowledgeable decisions.

A Cautionary Note

Magrann cautions to beware of diets that promise fast and easy weight loss or that cite nutrition information that is unsound or biased by financial gain.

On the other hand, according to Magrann, a sensible diet will:

--Teach good habits for permanent weight loss.

--Stress the importance of exercise.

--Be nutritionally balanced and will not eliminate any of the basic four food groups.

--Emphasize foods low in fat and high in nutritious carbohydrates such as fruits, vegetables, legumes and grain products.

--Recommend foods that are practical and economical.

--Recommend foods that the entire family can eat to avoid cooking separate meals.

Magrann also advises that the reader check the credentials of a person or persons giving the advice. "If the person is a registered dietitian, that means they have had a four-year degree from an accredited university and did additional training as an internship," she said. "They have also passed a registration test and have continuing education hours to their credit."

Conclusion

Comprehensive Guide to Health and Wellness" has taken you on a transformative journey through the realms of physical fitness, nutrition, and natural health remedies. It has armed you with knowledge, insights, and practical strategies to revitalize your life and embark on a path towards lasting well-being. As we conclude this journey, let's reflect on the key takeaways and the empowering message of this book.

Embrace the Power of Choice

Throughout these pages, you've learned that your health is not a predetermined fate but a result of the choices you make every day. The food you eat, the exercises you engage in, and the natural remedies you explore are all opportunities to invest in your well-being. "Fit For Life" emphasizes that you have the power to shape your health and destiny through informed, mindful choices.

Holistic Wellness is the Key

Wellness is not solely about a chiseled physique or a number on the scale; it's about nurturing your entire being—body, mind, and spirit. True health and vitality emerge when you embrace a holistic approach to wellness. This book has shown you that physical fitness, balanced nutrition, and natural health remedies are interconnected aspects of a harmonious life.

Personalization is Your Strength

Your journey to health and wellness is unique, and "Fit For Life" encourages you to embrace this individuality. Whether you're striving for improved fitness, weight management, stress reduction, or enhanced cognitive function, your path is your own. By customizing your wellness strategies to suit your needs and aspirations, you're setting yourself up for sustainable success.

A Lifelong Journey

The pursuit of fitness and wellness is not a destination but a lifelong journey. "Fit For Life" is not the end but a beginning—a guide that equips you with the knowledge and tools to navigate this journey. As you continue to explore, learn, and adapt, remember that the quest for well-being is an ongoing process filled with growth, discovery, and transformation.

Your Wellness Story

The story of your fitness and wellness is still being written. It's a narrative of resilience, triumphs, setbacks, and self-discovery. "Fit For Life" is but one chapter, a resource to consult whenever you seek guidance and inspiration. Your wellness story is about the choices you make, the actions you take, and the joy and vitality you cultivate along the way.

In conclusion, "Fit For Life" is not merely a book; it's a catalyst for positive change in your life. It invites you to embrace the power of choice, discover the beauty of holistic wellness, and embark on a personalized, lifelong journey towards a healthier, more vibrant you. As you close these pages and step forward into the world, carry with you the wisdom, confidence, and determination to be fit for life—today, tomorrow, and always.